Unlock the Power of Lycopene

*REDefining
Your Diet
for Optimum
Health*

by David Yeung, Ph.D.
and Venket Rao, Ph.D.

Foreword by Bob Watson, Businessman and
Former Major League Baseball All-Star and Front Office Executive

Introduction by Carolyn Aldigé, President and Founder
of the Cancer Research Foundation of America

Published by arpr, inc.

IMPORTANT NOTICE

The material contained in this book is for informational purposes only. It is not meant to function as a prescription or to substitute for the advice of a medical professional. Persons who have cancer, heart disease or other medical conditions should be guided by the direction and advice of their medical professionals. Good nutrition and sound dietary habits are not substitutes for treatment by a medical professional. Specifically, the consumption of lycopene and tomato products must not be substituted for the direction and advice of your medical professional. The authors and publisher disclaim and shall not be liable or responsible for any use, misuse or applications of this book to treat, diagnose or medicate a medical problem, disease or other condition.

UNLOCK THE POWER OF LYCOPENE
REDEFINING YOUR DIET FOR OPTIMUM HEALTH

Copyright © 2001 by arpr, inc.

All rights reserved. This book or any part herein may not be reproduced in any form without permission in writing from the copyright holder, except for brief quotations embodied in critical articles or reviews.

For information or inquiries address arpr, inc., 1420 Centre Avenue, Suite 2216, Pittsburgh, PA 15219 U.S.A.

ISBN: 0-9660991-7-6

For information or inquiries, visit www.lycopene.org

Printed in the United States of America
arpr, inc. paperback edition/April 2001

Library of Congress Cataloging-in-Publication Data

Yeung, David, 1939-
   Unlock the power of lycopene: redefining your diet for optimum health/ by David Yeung and Venket Rao.
    p. cm.
   Includes bibliographical references and index.
   ISBN 0-9660991-7-6 (pbk.)
    1. Tomatoes — Health aspects. 2. Lycopene — Health aspects. I. Rao, Venket, 1936- II. Title

QP144. V44 Y48   2001
613.2'8 – dc21   2001022845

TABLE OF CONTENTS

FOREWORD: A Few Words for Men From Businessman and Former Major League Baseball All-Star and Front Office Executive Bob Watson vii

INTRODUCTION: by Carolyn Aldigé xi

CHAPTER ONE: REDEFINING YOUR DIET
How Eating Right May Help Prevent Disease 1

CHAPTER TWO: TOMATO TRADITION
The Story of the Tomato, from the Aztecs to Today 9

CHAPTER THREE: TEAM TOMATO
Understanding the Tomato 14

CHAPTER FOUR: UNLOCK THE POWER
The Tomato's Many Health Benefits 21

CHAPTER FIVE: LESSONS IN LYCOPENE
A Scientific Look at This Powerful Antioxidant 30

CHAPTER SIX: NOW YOU'RE COOKING
Tasty Recipes for a Healthy Lifestyle 43

CHAPTER SEVEN: Q & A
Summing Up the Story of Lycopene 54

GLOSSARY 62

SOURCES 66

INDEX 72

ABOUT THE AUTHORS 80

Foreword

A Few Words for Men
From Businessman and Former Major League Baseball All-Star and Front Office Executive Bob Watson

Unlock the Power of Lycopene contains a wealth of information that should be of special interest to men: lycopene, a powerful antioxidant abundant in tomatoes, may help reduce the risk of many ailments, especially prostate cancer. As a survivor of that disease, I'd like to take this opportunity to shed some light on this feared ailment.

The prostate is a small gland, located beneath the bladder, that encircles the urethra. Cancer of the prostate is a serious health challenge. According to government reports, prostate cancer is the most commonly diagnosed form of cancer, other than skin cancer, among men in the United States and is second only to lung cancer as a cause of cancer-related deaths among men. Every year about 180,000 men are diagnosed with this disease, and more than 30,000 die from it.

Unfortunately, men hate to deal with health issues. That certainly was true of me. In April 1995, the last thing I was worrying about was my health. After 19 seasons as a big league ballplayer, I had climbed the management ladder and been named general manager of the Houston Astros, the first African-American man to become the top executive of a major league team. Baseball executives as well as the players are required to take a team physical, but I kept putting mine off. Finally the team doctor convinced me to come in for my checkup.

Foreword

I had no symptoms of any problems, no pain or any other warnings. But I had known two baseball scouts who had gotten PSA blood tests that had revealed prostate cancer. So I did ask for a PSA blood test, just in case. To my shock, the test indicated the possible presence of cancer. More tests and a biopsy confirmed that I had an aggressive form of prostate cancer. That was scary. All kinds of fears and thoughts raced through my mind. After evaluating all my options, I went ahead with surgery to remove the cancer in July of that year. It was a tough time, but the support of my wife, Carol, and everyone in the Astros organization was invaluable. The operation was a success, and I've been free of cancer for more than five years now.

The most important lesson for men is to see your doctor for regular physical examinations. Having a PSA test saved my life. Men don't like to go to the doctor, but it's essential. Your doctor can help you decide on the best measures to take, but he can't help if you don't see him.

Seeing the doctor is especially urgent if you are in a high-risk group: if you have a family member who had prostate cancer, if you are over 40, or if you are African-American. In fact, African-American men have the highest incidence of prostate cancer of any ethnic group. I'd like to get the message to men, and especially men in those groups, to see their doctors and get checked for prostate cancer.

You can fight back against prostate cancer. There are many treatment options available, and researchers continue to make progress in finding new and better ways to treat this disease. There is hope, and I'm living proof of that.

Another bit of good news can be found in this book: lycopene seems to reduce the risk of prostate cancer. For instance, an experiment at the Harvard School of Medicine studied the health of more than 47,000 men. The research showed that men who ate tomato products twice a week reduced their risk of getting a certain kind of prostate cancer by more than a third, compared to men who never ate tomato products.

So I urge you to read this book as a first step toward adopting a healthier lifestyle, including getting regular exercise and eating a balanced diet with plenty of fruits and vegetables. Then, if you haven't had a physical recently, get on the phone and call your doctor today!

Bob Watson

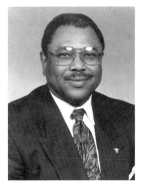

Bob Watson played Major League Baseball for 19 years and was named twice to the All-Star team. In his first full season as general manager of the New York Yankees, 1996, he engineered their first World Series victory since 1978. He was co-chairman of USA Baseball, the organization supporting the gold-medal-winning U.S. team at the 2000 Olympics in Sydney. He continues to serve as a consultant for Major League Baseball. Bob and his son Keith run Watson & Company, an entertainment finance consulting business. He also is a partner in Pinnacle Wealth Concepts, Ltd., a financial consulting firm.

INTRODUCTION

In the fight against cancer, we at the Cancer Research Foundation of America (CRFA) are always glad to get good news, and I think you'll find plenty of good news in *Unlock the Power of Lycopene*.

The good news begins with the growing consensus among medical professionals that a healthy diet, in conjunction with regular exercise and a healthy lifestyle, may play a significant role in fighting cancer. This consensus has not always existed. When CRFA opened its doors 15 years ago, mainstream science gave little thought to prevention. Since that day, thanks in part to the efforts of CRFA and the scientists it has supported, more and more people in the health field have recognized that all of us can take action to stay healthy.

Another bit of good news is that a healthy diet involves foods we already know and love. *Unlock the Power of Lycopene* will tell you why the tomatoes you love on your hamburgers or salads, or in spaghetti sauce or ketchup, are good for you, in addition to adding their bright color and zesty taste to your menus.

I think you will value the information provided in *Unlock the Power of Lycopene*. In Chapter One, you'll find out more about how the antioxidants in a healthy diet may help fight substances that cause disease. In Chapters Two and Three, you'll learn more about the tomato, from its origins in South America to its place in modern diets as one of our favorite sources of nutrition.

Chapter Four will showcase many of the tomato's health benefits. Chapter Five will tell you more about lycopene. It is the pigment that makes tomatoes red, and it is also a powerful antioxidant that holds promise as a cancer fighter. Much research remains to be done, but we at CRFA are very hopeful that future research on lycopene, and other natural substances, will help us fight cancer.

Chapter Six will offer you some delightful recipes, and Chapter Seven will provide a question-and-answer session about lycopene and its great potential.

Unlock the Power of Lycopene will offer you both vital information about lycopene and fun facts about the tomato. I truly hope that it will inspire you to add more tomatoes and other fruits and vegetables to your meals, as a step toward enjoying a healthy diet and lifestyle. We at CRFA are moving forward with our drive to expand research and education to prevent cancer. We'd love to know that people like you are joining us in the fight — especially since one simple step you can take is to add delicious tomatoes and processed tomato products to your diet!

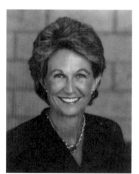

Carolyn Aldigé

Carolyn Aldigé founded the Cancer Research Foundation of America (CRFA) in 1985 as a national, nonprofit health foundation with a single mission: the prevention of cancer through scientific research and education. CRFA has provided funding to more than 200 scientists at more than 100 leading academic institutions.

CHAPTER ONE

REDefining Your Diet

How Eating Right May Help Prevent Disease

Scientists are gathering more and more information about the potential health benefits of lycopene, a substance that makes tomatoes red and may help prevent many diseases. To understand lycopene, we need to look first at the growing evidence that diet plays a crucial role in fighting disease.

We live in an age of medical miracles — but some of the most powerful aids to your health can be found in your garden or in the processed foods in your refrigerator. Even as doctors build high-tech devices and discover powerful new drugs, other researchers are finding more and more evidence that a healthy lifestyle, with a diet rich in fruits and vegetables, may be able to prevent and even fight serious diseases.

That's right: a dinner of spaghetti with marinara sauce and a side of broccoli might be a step forward in keeping your heart and blood vessels healthy; adding an orange and a glass of tomato juice to your lunch might be part of a healthy lifestyle that can help you fight cancer.

That's because diet, combined with other lifestyle habits, may play a major role in preventing disease. You may have heard of the Mediterranean diet, which is rich in fruits, vegetables, grains, and olive oil and low in saturated fat. Research has shown that such a diet may help cut the risk of heart disease. Much research is showing that similar health benefits are associated with other healthy diets.

By some estimates, a better diet combined with a healthier lifestyle (such as getting regular exercise) could cut the number of cancer cases by one-third and also might reduce the number of heart attacks.

Although health experts agree that much serious scientific work remains to be done in this vital and complex subject, diet and other lifestyle factors may play a role in dozens of diseases, including many of the deadliest. Today a number of major American health organizations are on record as saying that a balanced diet with plenty of fruits and vegetables, as part of a healthy

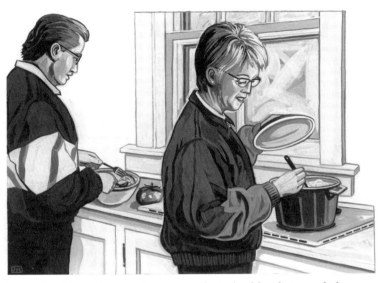

A growing body of research suggests that a healthy diet may help prevent disease.

lifestyle that includes regular exercise and other common sense steps, seems to be linked to a reduced risk of disease. These organizations include:

- The American Cancer Society
- The U.S. Department of Health and Human Services
- The National Cancer Institute
- The U.S. Food and Drug Administration
- The American Heart Association
- The American Medical Association

"You are what you eat," many parents have told their children. And, as in so many other things, they were right! The difference today is that scientists are discovering additional ways fruits and vegetables help fight disease. Scientists are still researching those benefits, and they don't have all the answers yet. But in the meantime, we can take advantage of what we do know and enjoy the fruits and vegetables we have always loved. One way to think of it is to brighten your plate with delicious fruits and vegetables. One of the best is the tomato. When you "REDefine" your diet, all you have to do is add the bright red of the tomato to your table. This can be in salads, juices, sauces, and literally hundreds of other dishes and recipes.

To understand why, we need to understand "functional foods."

DISEASE-FIGHTING FOODS

Functional foods are broadly defined as foods that, in addition to meeting nutritional needs, may supply other health benefits. One example of a functional food is calcium-fortified orange juice. The calcium is thought to be of benefit in preventing osteoporosis. However, many foods might be considered "functional foods." For example, regular orange juice is full of Vitamin C, and that in itself has health benefits. There is some evidence that some functional foods may help fight four of the leading causes of death: cancer, diabetes, cardiovascular disease and high blood pressure.

Functional foods also may play a role in fighting depression, arthritis, osteoporosis and other diseases.

Fruits and vegetables are natural functional foods because they are full of phytochemicals, a word that simply means "plant chemicals." Phytochemicals are natural plant substances that perform a number of functions, including protecting some plants from disease. Scientific research suggests that some phytochemicals also may help protect our bodies from disease. There are thousands of phytochemicals, some of which have been used for hundreds of years as medicines, such as quinine for malaria and digitalis for heart conditions.

Scientists have especially studied one group of phytochemicals: the antioxidants. Antioxidants may play a role in fighting many diseases, including cancer, heart disease, age-related macular degeneration, diabetes and osteoporosis. If we take a close look at antioxidants, we'll understand how tomatoes and other fruits and vegetables might be able to help fight disease.

Antioxidants to the Rescue

Some scientists think that antioxidants may protect your health by fighting substances in your body called free radicals. Free radicals are unstable molecules produced, for example, when your body burns (oxidizes) food. Like a car's engine burning gasoline and producing exhaust and pollution, this process produces a kind of internal pollution: free radicals. Indeed, pollution, smoking and other environmental factors can create more free radicals in our bodies.

Another way to think about oxidation is to understand that it is the same process that makes iron rust and fruit turn brown. It doesn't take much to see that free radicals do the same kind of damage to the cells in your body. You might think of free radicals as pirates roaming the sea, looking for ships to capture and plunder, often sinking them in the process. In this case, the plundered ships are some of the most vital cells in your body.

Moreover, when a free radical attacks another molecule, it turns that molecule into a free radical, setting off a chain reaction creating more and more free radicals, which in turn damage more cells. Many scientists think this cell damage may trigger a host of diseases including cancer and heart disease.

Fortunately, as their name suggests, antioxidants protect us from oxidative damage. Antioxidants sometimes act like bodyguards protecting cells; other antioxidants are the body's peacemakers, helping free radicals settle down before they can do damage. Some of the best known are Vitamin A, Vitamin C, Vitamin E and beta-carotene.

One of the best reasons for adding red to your diet is that tomatoes are full of one of the most powerful antioxidants — lycopene. Because lycopene is about twice as powerful an antioxidant as beta-carotene, it has tremendous potential as a disease-fighter.

Lycopene may help reduce the risk of cancer. In one experiment, researchers at the Harvard School of Medicine studied the health of 47,894 men. The research showed that consuming tomato products twice a week, as opposed to never, was associated with a reduced risk of prostate cancer of up to 34 percent.

Lycopene also may help fight heart disease. A research project at the University of North Carolina reviewed the current evidence and summarized it by saying that much research suggests lycopene may help fight cardiovascular disease. For example, a university scientist studied diets in 10 European nations and found that people who had the highest lycopene consumption had half the risk of heart attacks.

Tomatoes and processed tomato products also are full of other valuable substances, including Vitamin A and Vitamin C. Moreover, you don't need to do any scientific experiments to know that vegetables and fruits are far tastier and much more fun to eat than a pill. Perhaps that's the bottom line: you can't go wrong by eating plenty of fruits and vegetables, and one way to do that is to REDefine your diet by adding tomatoes or processed tomato products. We'll tell you more about the many health benefits of the tomato in Chapters Four and Five, but let's turn now to the tomato itself. What we'll learn will help us appreciate this handy, nutritious and tasty vegetable ... or is it a fruit?

CHAPTER TWO

TOMATO TRADITION

THE STORY OF THE TOMATO, FROM THE AZTECS TO TODAY

Today the tomato is one of our favorite sources of nutrition — but it faced a tough fight to be accepted on menus in the United States, Canada, Great Britain, much of northern Europe and Asia.

The tomato originated in the Andes Mountains in South America and was first domesticated in Mexico by the Aztec people. The word "tomato" seems to be derived from the Aztec word "tomatl." After the Spanish conquered Mexico in the early 1500s, they introduced it to southern Europe, where it quickly became popular. The Italians may have called it "pomodoro" — golden apple — perhaps because the first tomatoes often were yellow. But others say that the Italian name originally was "poma amoris," meaning "apple of love." The French also called it the apple of love, "pomme d'amour." This name may have been prompted by the heart shape of many tomatoes of that era and gave rise to the legend that the tomato was an aphrodisiac.

The tomato received a much chillier reception in colder climates, however. In parts of the United States, Canada and Great Britain, it often was called the "wolf peach." This rather unappealing name reflects the poor reputation of the tomato in those countries and throughout much of northern Europe. Many people even thought tomatoes were poisonous. This belief may have sprung from the fact that the tomato is related to poisonous plants such as belladonna and nightshade, and indeed vines and leaves of the tomato plant can be poisonous. Whatever the reason, for many years it was grown only as a decorative plant in much of North America and northern Europe.

Another reason, perhaps, for the reluctance of people in northern countries to eat tomatoes was that most diets in those regions were bland, both in taste and color. In the era before refrigeration and mass transportation, fresh fruits and vegetables were available only for short portions of the year. People used to a diet of starches and meat were slow to realize the culinary potential of the tomato's vibrant red color and resonant flavor. Nevertheless, it slowly made inroads. Thomas Jefferson grew them at his farm at Monticello as early as 1781 as a decorative plant. In the early 1800s it began to gain some cautious acceptance in the United States.

A story illustrates the process. In Salem, N.J., about 1822, amateur horticulturist Robert Gibbon Johnson vowed to eat tomatoes on the steps of the courthouse. His own physician warned him he would "foam and froth at the mouth ... double over with appendicitis ... if [the] 'wolf peach' is too ripe and warmed by the sun ... exposing himself to brain fever." A crowd gathered to watch this horrific spectacle. Johnson went ahead and

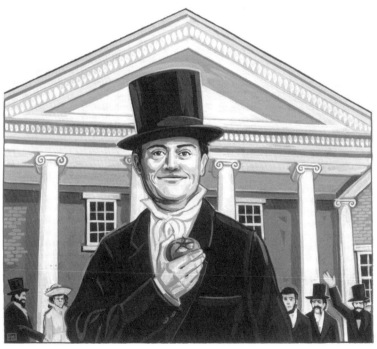

By daring to eat a tomato, Robert Gibbon Johnson inspired Americans to accept tomatoes as a food.

ate tomatoes from his garden. To the surprise of the townsfolk, he displayed obvious relish for the juicy red vegetables and suffered no evident side effects. From Salem the word spread: tomatoes were not only safe, they were delicious — or so the story goes.

In any event, by the middle of the 19th century the tomato had become widely accepted in the United States and the rest of the world. One factor was the growing popularity of tomato ketchup. Ketchup has been around for centuries, though its precise origins are in dispute. It may have been created in Asia; some experts have speculated the word "ketchup" was originally a Malay word, "kitjap." At first ketchup meant any of a wide array of sauces, including some made from walnuts, beans or anchovies. With the growing popularity of the tomato, tomato ketchup became a favorite way to add the taste and color of tomatoes to meals year-round.

Farmers and horticulturists rapidly developed the red, round tomato we see most often in our supermarkets today. In 1949, the first hybrid tomatoes appeared, aiding tomato production. For instance, in the 1960s the development of hardy breeds of tomatoes, along with the refinement of tomato-harvesting machines, aided the cultivation of processing tomatoes. The tomato crop is, after the potato crop, the most important commercial vegetable product in the United States, both in terms of how many tomatoes are grown and how many tomatoes and tomato products are consumed. It also is, according to some experts, the biggest contributor of nutrients to the American diet.

The situation is similar in other countries. Tomatoes now are grown virtually throughout the world and have revolutionized diets across the globe. The tomato has made its biggest mark in Italian, Spanish and Mexican cooking, but cooks everywhere have found it to be versatile and tasty. You could easily have a different tomato-based recipe every day of the year, with plenty left over. The tomato has found a role in an almost unlimited number of casseroles, stews and other main dishes, from shrimp jambalaya to tomato chow mein to tomato cake, not to mention a multitude of sauces and dressings.

But what lies behind its popularity? Let's find out.

CHAPTER THREE

TEAM TOMATO

UNDERSTANDING THE TOMATO

A look at the tomato itself will help us understand why it is such a popular source of nutrition.

Tomatoes answer to the scientific name of Lycopersicon esculentum, which roughly translates as "edible wolf peach," recalling the days it was eyed with suspicion. The tomato indeed is related to the poisonous nightshade plants, and also is part of the larger Solanaceae family, which includes potatoes, eggplant, and cayenne and tabasco peppers.

Tomatoes and tomato sauces are packed with nutrients, with little fat and no cholesterol. For example, 100 grams of tomato sauce has 30 calories, 1.3 grams of protein, 7 grams of carbohydrates and a little more than a gram of fiber.

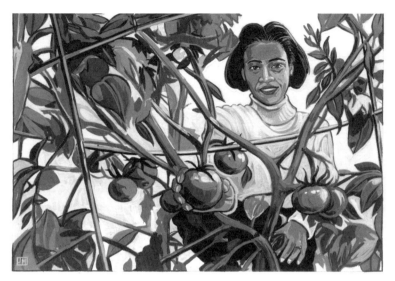

More than nine out of 10 home gardens in the United States include tomatoes.

VARIETIES

Let's look at the many different kinds of tomatoes and tomato plants.

Size. Tomatoes generally range in size from three-quarters of an inch in diameter and a quarter of an ounce in weight to six inches in diameter and two pounds, but some are much bigger. The biggest tomato on record was a seven-pound behemoth grown in Oklahoma.

Color. Tomatoes range in hue from white to red to purple, including green, yellow and orange. The lighter colors generally have a milder flavor. One note: only red tomatoes have lycopene, because lycopene is the red pigment that gives them their color.

Determinate and indeterminate plants. "Determinate" tomato plants are rather compact bushes that grow to a certain size and then stop, with their tomatoes reaching maturity at roughly the same time. "Indeterminate" tomato plants, or vines, keep growing until the frost (or extreme heat in warmer climates) kills them.

Store tomatoes and processing tomatoes. Store (fresh market) tomatoes are picked when they are green, because they need to ripen during the trip to market to have the best flavor. They also are picked by hand because they must be picked at just the right stage in the ripening process and then must arrive on the shelves in perfect condition.

To give consumers the best prices and quality for sauces and ketchup, processing tomatoes must be harvested in the most efficient manner possible, and this means that the tomatoes themselves need to be different. First of all, they must be picked together at the peak of ripeness, then processed within a few hours of ripening. This means that they are grown on determinate plants that have been specially bred so that the tomatoes ripen at about the same time. Efficiency requires machine harvesting and rapid transportation, so growers have developed hardy tomatoes that can withstand being picked by machines and not be crushed when transported at the bottom of 25,000-pound truckloads, yet still have all the taste and nutrition you expect in tomato products.

Shape. The five main shapes are, in order of size, cherry, plum, pear, standard and beefsteak.

Maturity date. This is the number of days from the date of planting to the time when they can be expected to be ripe.

Flavor. Studies have shown that a substance called furenol, which develops during the ripening process, is the main source of the tomato's flavor. That is why tomatoes need to ripen to present the best taste. Also, there isn't much difference in the acidity of most kinds of tomatoes. Tomatoes that taste "less acidic" really just have more natural sugar.

The popular varieties of garden tomatoes alone

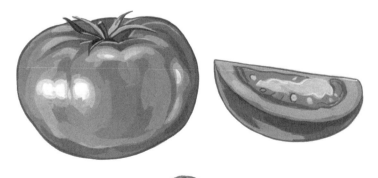

number in the hundreds. To give you an idea of the tomato's many colors, sizes and flavors, here are names of just a few of the popular tomato varieties:

Celebrity Champion	Better Boy	Bucks County
Dona	Delicious	French Rose
Early Girl	Fourth of July	Red Star
Fantastic	Tumbler	Mortgage Lifter
Golden Nugget	Medina	Lemon Boy
Jubilee	Heatwave II	Good 'n Early
Mr. Stripey	Celebrity	Garden Peach
Siberia	Red Satin	Small Fry
Sun Gold	Sweet Tangerine	Big Beef
Sweet Million	Saladette Ensalada	Best Boy
Top Sirloin	Green Grape	

FRUIT OR VEGETABLE?

There's one more way of describing tomatoes that occasionally sparks disputes: are they fruits or vegetables?

If you're like most people, you think of tomatoes as vegetables. After all, in a salad they are eaten with lettuce, green pepper, onions and other vegetables; we cook tomatoes along with other vegetables in sauces or casseroles. But if you talked to a botanist, he or she might insist that the tomato is a fruit. What's the answer? In a way, the answer is "both of the above."

In botanical terms, the tomato itself is a fruit, because a fruit is considered to be any sweet pulp containing a seed or seeds. A horticulturist, however, would say the tomato plant is a vegetable plant. That is because most "fruits" are grown on trees: think of apple, peach or cherry trees. But the tomato plant is a vine or a bush, like most of the plants you'll see in a typical vegetable garden.

In the United States, the argument has been settled by the highest court in the land. In 1893 the U.S. Supreme Court ruled on a lawsuit on that very question because at the time vegetables were subject to a tariff and fruits were not. "Botanically speaking," the Court ruled, "tomatoes are the fruit of a vine, just as are cucumbers, squashes, beans and peas. But in the common language of the people, whether sellers or consumers of provisions, all these are vegetables which are grown in kitchen gardens, and which, whether eaten cooked or raw, are, like potatoes, carrots, parsnips, turnips, beets, cauliflower, cabbage, celery, and lettuce, usually served at dinner in, with, or after the soup, fish, or meats which constitute the principal part of the repast, and not, like fruits generally, as dessert."

Today many people follow the Court's reasoning and call the tomato a vegetable.

Popularity

Although tomato plants generally require warm weather and lots of sunlight, they are adaptable and vigorous. This is shown by the fact that, of the nearly 30 million Americans who have gardens, perhaps as many as 95 percent of them grow tomatoes, making it the most popular home-garden vegetable in the United States. The tomato has been just as enthusiastically received in other nations, though in colder climates it usually is grown in greenhouses.

Thanks to the tomato's own adaptability, varieties, many uses, and modern development, it has become very popular. Americans consume an average of more than 90 pounds of tomatoes every year for every man, woman and child in the nation, with about 17 pounds of that as fresh tomatoes, and the rest as processed tomato products. To meet this demand, American farmers in 1999 grew more than 1.7 million tons of fresh-market tomatoes and more than 12.8 million tons of processing tomatoes.

Let's turn now to another source of the tomato's popularity in our health-conscious age: its many nutrients.

CHAPTER FOUR

Unlock the Power

The Tomato's Many Health Benefits

Regardless of whether the tomato is called a fruit or vegetable, it is an important component in the North American diet. As we saw in Chapter One, dietitians recommend that we choose sensibly in what we eat and stay physically active. To achieve a healthy lifestyle we are asked to:

- Choose a diet that is low in saturated fat and cholesterol, and moderate in total fat.
- Choose beverages and foods to moderate your intake of sugars.
- Choose and prepare foods with less salt.
- If you drink alcoholic beverages, do so in moderation.

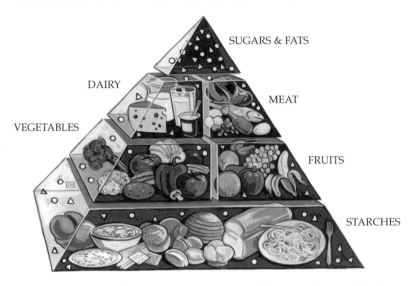

The Food Pyramid illustrates the importance of fruits and vegetables in the well-balanced diet.

To ensure that we get all the essential nutrients in the right amounts, nutrition experts suggest we follow the well-known Food Pyramid as a starting point.

Fruits and vegetables are key elements of our daily diets. Regular consumption of fruits and vegetables (five to nine servings per day) may help to reduce the risk of certain chronic diseases. Fruits and vegetables are very good sources of vitamins, minerals and fiber.

Tomatoes contain important substances that are referred to as functional components, which are natural substances in conventional or traditional foods that exert a physiological or health benefit together with basic nutrition. An example is the antioxidants found in brightly colored fruit and green leafy vegetables.

Tomato Essence

Tomatoes are an important part of the vegetable food group, and are the second most consumed vegetable in North America. The tomato is a treasure of nutrients, including Vitamin C, Vitamin A, potassium, folic acid, and others. In 100 grams of raw tomato there are 1,000 international units of Vitamin A, 60 micrograms of Vitamin B1, 40 micrograms of Vitamin B2, 28 micrograms of folic acid, 22 milligrams of Vitamin C, 1.2 milligrams of Vitamin E, 290 milligrams of potassium, 21 milligrams of calcium, and 14 milligrams of magnesium.

Processed tomatoes have higher levels of the nutrients simply because the vegetable is concentrated. Because of the volume of tomatoes and tomato products that North Americans customarily eat, tomatoes have been ranked No. 1 in the total amount of nutrients they contribute to our diet. (See chart on page 25.)

The Tomato "C"

Many of us do not realize that tomatoes contribute the second highest amount of Vitamin C in our diets in

North America. (Citrus fruits, such as oranges, provide the most.) Vitamin C has long been known to prevent scurvy, a scourge among our ancestors when fruits and vegetables were not always available. Scurvy is a condition that is characterized by bleeding gums and soreness in the joints.

Vitamin C also is a powerful antioxidant. In nature, it helps retain the color and freshness of fruits and vegetables. In the human body, it may prevent certain degenerative diseases. It is believed to prevent and to reduce the duration of the common cold. Vitamin C also has the ability to enhance the absorption of important nutrients such as iron and zinc.

ALL THE BETTER TO SEE YOU WITH — VITAMIN A

Tomato consumption is the fourth most important source of Vitamin A in our diets. This is because of the high levels of beta-carotene, which is converted to Vitamin A in our bodies.

Vitamin A is important for vision. A lack of Vitamin A can lead to night blindness, which is the inability of our eyes to adapt from bright light to darkness. Extreme deprivation of Vitamin A can lead to total blindness.

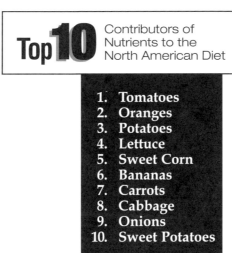

Charles, M. R., "The Tomato," *Scientific American*, 1978, 239:76-87

Vitamin A also is very important for the maintenance of the skin and tissue lining, including that of the eye. Vitamin A is important for immune functions and, therefore, for the prevention of infections. A lack of the vitamin can result in a greater risk for cancer of the lungs and other organs where the mucous lining becomes affected.

POTASSIUM POWER

Potassium is an essential nutrient that is important for normal health maintenance and growth. Tomatoes contribute the ninth highest amount of potassium in our diets.

In the body, potassium, as an electrolyte, is necessary for controlling acid-base balance, movement of nutrients across the cell membranes, nerve conduction and muscle contraction. A deficiency of potassium can result in cramps, muscle weakness, mental confusion, apathy, anorexia and coma. For athletes involved in endurance events, who lose potassium when they sweat, it is important that they have ample potassium in their bodies. The level can be bolstered before or replaced during and after performance by eating foods or drinking fluids high in potassium.

The potassium in tomatoes, as well as the calcium and the magnesium, also may play a role in reducing high blood pressure.

OTHER NUTRIENTS

Besides the nutrients mentioned above, tomato consumption delivers many other important vitamins and minerals. These include folic acid and some of the other B vitamins.

In recent years, nutritionists have identified the importance of folic acid for pregnant women. Intake of adequate levels of folic acid prior to and in early gestation may reduce the risk of neural tube defects in the newborn. Furthermore, older individuals who have unusually high levels of homocysteine, an amino acid, in the blood, may be more prone to heart disease. Regular intake of high levels of folic acid may reduce the amount of homocysteine in the bloodstream, thus reducing the risk of heart disease. In both situations, the suggested dietary intake of folic acid is 40 micrograms per day. This easily can be achieved by regularly eating vegetables such as tomatoes and spinach that are high in this nutrient. Nevertheless, folic acid supplements may be recommended for pregnant women or women who may become pregnant, so a doctor's advice should be sought regarding the adequacy of folic acid intake in the diet.

FUNCTIONAL COMPONENTS

Tomatoes are excellent sources of a good number of functional components. Scientists now are beginning to unravel some of these components. Many of these functional components have antioxidative or hormonal properties. Others may promote the growth of organ tissues or biologically healthy bacteria in the intestinal tract. Functional components can be found in cruciferous vegetables, brightly colored fruits and vegetables, fish, red wine, garlic, green tea, soybeans, whole grains and bran. Tomatoes are the highest sources of the functional components lycopene and oligosaccharides in North American diets.

Lycopene is the carotenoid that gives the tomato its typical red color. One of the small numbers of carotenoids that cannot be converted to Vitamin A, lycopene is one of the most powerful antioxidants among the carotenoids. In the body, free radicals constantly attack body lipids (fats), such as cholesterol, resulting in heart disease. They also can attack the genetic materials (DNA) and damage cells, causing cancers and other dreaded chronic diseases. Available antioxidants from the diet can help to ward off the damaging effects of antioxidants by intercepting them before they can do harm.

Lycopene has been shown to be an antioxidant that can possibly reduce the risk of heart disease, certain types of cancer, age-related macular degeneration and diabetes (as will be discussed in the following chapter).

Oligosaccharides are carbohydrates that are not broken down by the intestinal enzymes. However, they serve as nourishment for the bacteria in the colon that help us digest food.

In addition to lycopene and oligosaccharides, the tomato contains a number of other carotenoids that may work in concert with lycopene as antioxidants. There are other unknown components in tomatoes that are functional. Preliminary research has shown that the yellow fluid surrounding the seeds might be able to, in some unknown way, prevent blood clots and cardiovascular disease.

Furthermore, the carbohydrate-binding protein in tomatoes has the highest agglutination activity of any fruit. Agglutination is the process of binding certain bacteria or foreign cells together, which is one way the body fights bacteria. It may be beneficial against inflammatory intestinal diseases and boost immunity.

Unlocking the Magic

The level of nutrients is highest during ripening of vegetables. The redder the tomato, the higher the level of lycopene.

Heat processing helps to unlock the lycopene, making it more available for absorption. The process converts the structure of lycopene to a form that can be more easily absorbed in the small intestines. Furthermore, processing breaks down the cell structure of the tomato, thereby releasing more of the lycopene. Processing also concentrates the product and therefore the lycopene.

Consumption of processed tomato products in a meal that has a small amount of fat also will enhance its absorption. Lycopene dissolves in fat, hence the importance of a small amount of dietary fat in the digestive process.

Now let's find out in more depth what science tells us about lycopene.

CHAPTER FIVE

LESSONS IN LYCOPENE

A SCIENTIFIC LOOK AT THIS POWERFUL ANTIOXIDANT

As we've learned so far, lycopene, in its role as an antioxidant, may help fight disease. Free radicals interact with critical cellular components such as lipids (fats), proteins and DNA, causing oxidative damage leading to diseases. Antioxidants may reduce the effects of oxidative damage, as we discussed briefly in Chapter One.

Lycopene is a natural red pigment belonging to the carotenoid family that is produced by plants and some micro-organisms but not by animals and humans. Red fruits and vegetables such as tomatoes, watermelons, pink guava, and pink grapefruit are some of the major sources of dietary lycopene. In North America, more than 85 percent of the dietary lycopene is derived from tomatoes and tomato-based products.

In chemical terms, lycopene has a large number of "double bonds." These are chemical bonds in which two pairs of electrons are shared by two atoms in a molecule. This may be the basis of lycopene's power in fighting free radicals. Free radicals lack an electron, and they cause damage by grabbing electrons away from other molecules. Because it has many double bonds, lycopene is more able to donate an electron to free radicals, taming them and, in the process, protecting the body.

Indeed, lycopene is one of the most powerful antioxidants. For comparison, you may have read a lot about the antioxidant beta-carotene, but lycopene has twice the power of beta-carotene to "quench" free radicals, and thus fight disease.

Lycopene, to be beneficial in the prevention of chronic diseases, must first be absorbed and then maintain its antioxidant properties in the body. Several factors influence the absorption and hence the bioavailability of lycopene. For instance, studies have shown that lycopene is absorbed more efficiently from heat-processed tomato products than it is from fresh tomatoes. This is because lycopene is bound into the tomato's cell structure, and when released from that structure during processing it becomes more available. The presence of fats also facilitates the absorption of lycopene.

Another important factor is the chemical form of lycopene present in tomatoes. Recent studies have shown that processing tomatoes changes their lycopene into a form that is more easily absorbed by the body.

The presence of other dietary components such as beta-carotene and Vitamin E also may influence the absorption of lycopene. Recent studies have shown that ingesting cooked tomato juice in an oil medium increased the level of lycopene in the blood by three-fold compared to an equivalent amount of unprocessed juice. In another study, lycopene from tomato paste was shown to be more bioavailable than lycopene from fresh tomatoes.

Following the absorption of dietary lycopene, it is distributed throughout the body to various organs. Some organs, such as the prostate, liver, adrenal gland and testes, have been shown to contain much higher levels of lycopene, suggesting the presence of specialized transport mechanisms in these organs.

The main supporting evidence for the role of lycopene in disease prevention comes from three kinds of scientific studies:

- Tissue culture studies that investigate how cells develop
- Laboratory study of animals
- Epidemiological studies

These studies are continuing to provide a great deal of evidence for the health benefits of lycopene. Let us look first at how lycopene might fight cancer.

Cancer Fighter

Cancer is a multistage disease in which a normal cell undergoes genetic alteration due to DNA damage. This stage is referred to as the "initiation" stage. The initiated cells then proliferate under certain conditions. The stage in which cells proliferate is then followed by a "progression" stage. Eventually, malignant primary tumors are formed that undergo metastasis and spread throughout the body.

Lycopene can play an important role in fighting this process. As a potent antioxidant, it can prevent oxidative damage of the DNA and prevent the progression of cancer at its early stage. It also can battle cancer by preventing cell proliferation typical of cancer, and also by restricting the growth of tumor cells.

Several studies have shown that the presence of lycopene can prevent the growth of several cancer cell lines. Similarly, animal studies also have demonstrated that the presence of lycopene in the diet can prevent spontaneous and chemically induced cancers.

However, the main evidence in support of the role of lycopene in the prevention of cancer comes from epidemiological studies, which examine the health of large groups of people over long periods of time. For example, researchers have studied the diet and health of people in the Mediterranean countries, whose diets often include more vegetables, olive oil and tomatoes. This Mediterranean diet has been suggested as a possible cause for the lower cancer rates in that region. Other studies have shown that a high intake of tomatoes resulted in lower incidence of digestive tract cancers and a 50 percent reduction in rates of death from cancers at all sites in an elderly U.S. population.

Consider another recent scientific study of a large group of people. It showed that the higher the level of lycopene in their blood and tissue, the less risk they ran of suffering breast or prostate cancer. The same study found no such effect with the other carotenoids.

In another report summing up 72 epidemiological studies, tomato-based products and lycopene were evaluated with respect to the incidence of cancers. Almost 80 percent of the studies reviewed showed that for the people studied, the higher the amount of lycopene in the bloodstream, or the more tomatoes and tomato products eaten, the less risk those people had of suffering several types of cancer. None of the studies showed any adverse effects to consuming tomatoes and tomato products.

PROSTATE CANCER

The main focus of lycopene and cancer research so far has been in the area of prostate cancer.

Another study discovered an inverse relationship between the estimated intake of lycopene from various tomato products and the risk of prostate cancer. That is, the more tomato products men consumed, the less likely it was that they suffered from prostate cancer. None of the other carotenoids demonstrated a similar relationship. In this study, a reduction in the risk of prostate cancer of almost 35 percent was observed for men who consumed 10 or more servings of tomato products per week. Interestingly, the protective effect of lycopene was more pronounced with advanced or aggressive stages of prostate cancer.

Lycopene Content in Popular Foods and Products*	
Product	Lycopene (mg/100 g)
Tomato Paste	42.2
Spaghetti Sauce	21.9
Chili Sauce	19.5
Seafood Sauce	17.0
Tomato Ketchup	15.9
Tomato Sauce	14.1
Tomato Juice	9.5
Tomato Soup (Condensed)	7.2
Watermelon	4.0
Pink Grapefruit	4.0
Raw Tomato	3.0

*Assuming equal quantities consumed.

Source: www.lycopene.org/content/index.html

Ingesting lycopene in the form of tomato juice and sauce was shown in a recent study to significantly increase lycopene levels in the blood and reduce oxidative stress. In another study, blood and tissue levels of lycopene in prostate cancer patients were shown to be significantly lower than their age-matched control subjects. When the prostate cancer patients ingested 50 milligrams of lycopene daily for four weeks in the form of tomato juice, there was a significant increase in their serum lycopene levels and a corresponding decrease in the signs of oxidation. The study also showed that low levels of lycopene in the bloodstream often were associated with high PSA (prostate specific antigen) levels. This is important because high PSA levels often are a sign of prostate cancer.

Similar results also were shown in another study with prostate cancer patients. In this study a regression of the tumor also was observed.

The emerging concepts that explain the role of lycopene in cancer prevention include:
- Oxidative stress is related to cancer risk.
- Antioxidants mitigate the effect of oxidative damage.
- Dietary lycopene is readily absorbed and acts as an antioxidant to prevent oxidative damage of lipids, protein and DNA, thereby possibly lowering the risk of cancer.
- In addition to the antioxidant effects of lycopene, some studies suggest it also may prevent the proliferation of cancer cells and enhance the immune response.

HEART PROTECTOR

Free radicals also cause oxidation of low-density lipoproteins (LDL), which function as the carriers of cholesterol in the bloodstream. This damage to LDL now is recognized as an important early step in the development of atherosclerosis. Dietary antioxidants such as lycopene may slow the progression of atherosclerosis because of their ability to inhibit oxidative damage.

Several epidemiological studies now have demonstrated that consuming tomatoes and tomato products containing lycopene reduces the risk of cardiovascular disease. In a study in which subjects were recruited from 10 European countries, the relationship between adipose tissue antioxidant levels and heart attacks was examined. After adjusting for several dietary variables, only the level of lycopene in the blood was shown to protect against cardiovascular disease.

Indirect evidence for the beneficial role of carotenoids, including lycopene, was provided in a study in which low levels of these antioxidants were shown to increase the risk of subsequent heart attacks in the high-risk population of cigarette smokers. Similarly, in another study comparing populations with different rates of coronary artery disease, lower blood lycopene levels were found to be associated with increased risk for, and death from, the disease.

Consider another study. In a small clinical trial involving six male subjects, dietary supplementation of lycopene at the level of 60 milligrams per day for three months was shown to reduce plasma LDL levels by 14 percent. This suggests that lycopene may be a moderate agent in reducing cholesterol.

Although the epidemiological evidence for the role of

lycopene in the prevention of cardiovascular disease is persuasive, it remains to be proven using well-controlled clinical intervention studies in populations at high risk for cardiovascular disease. It also is not clear as to the levels of lycopene intake that would be required to provide protection against the risk of heart disease.

OTHER DISEASES

Scientists across the world are now investigating how lycopene might help prevent other diseases and ailments. There is evidence that lycopene might help prevent age-related macular degeneration (ARMD), a disease that can

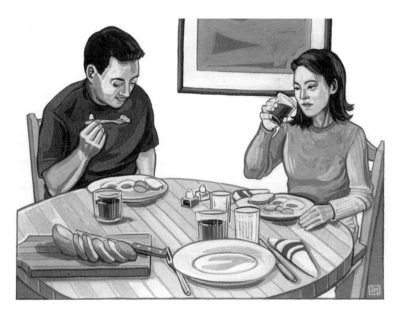

There are hundreds of dishes and foods with tomatoes and tomato products that can add lycopene to your meals.

lead to blindness. For example, a study at the University of Wisconsin showed that people with the lowest level of lycopene in their bloodstream were twice as likely to get ARMD as the other people who were studied.

It also is recognized that chronic diseases such as osteoporosis and diabetes are related to oxidative damage. Some studies have been performed investigating the effectiveness of lycopene in reducing the risk of these diseases.

In a major study in the United States, scientists discovered that the amounts of lycopene and beta-carotene were on average highest in people with normal glucose tolerance, slightly lower in people with impaired glucose tolerance, and lowest in people with newly diagnosed diabetes.

Other studies investigated the effect of lycopene on the activity of bone cells. Rodent osteoclast cells, which are responsible for the breakdown and resorption of bone material, were incubated in the presence of different concentrations of lycopene and their activity estimated. Results indicated that lycopene might inhibit osteoclast cell activity. These preliminary results perhaps suggest a beneficial role for lycopene in the prevention of osteoporosis.

Research is ongoing, but there is a great deal of

evidence that lycopene has many health benefits. Remember, however, that good nutrition, including consumption of tomato products, is not a substitute for medical advice and treatment. The basic message is simply this: something as delicious as tomato products may also be good for you. At this point, you may well agree that it would be a good idea to add a splash of bright red tomato products to your diet. But how much do you need?

Lycopene in Your Daily Diet

In one study, when healthy people consumed lycopene in the range of 25 to 150 milligrams daily in the form of tomato products and lycopene capsules for a week, a significant increase in the level of lycopene in their blood and a reduction in indications of oxidation were observed at all levels of intake.

A recently completed study evaluated the effect of ingesting low levels of lycopene on its absorption and antioxidant properties. Lycopene at the levels of 5, 10 and 20 milligrams was ingested by healthy people in the form of ketchup for a period of two weeks. Once again, a significant increase in serum lycopene levels and a reduction in lipid oxidation were observed at all levels of lycopene intake. The recommended daily intake level of lycopene therefore can be revised to 5 to 10 milligrams.

This level of dietary lycopene can help maintain levels of lycopene to deal with normal oxidative stress. The recommended level of lycopene intake is easily achievable by consuming a variety of tomato products. A tablespoon of ketchup, for example, supplies 2.7 milligrams of lycopene. (See chart on page 36.)

As of now, recommendations of daily lycopene intake levels in populations at high risk for cancer, cardiovascular disease and other chronic diseases cannot be established. Future studies must be undertaken with these populations to see if larger daily doses of lycopene are beneficial for people at risk for those diseases.

THE BOTTOM LINE

There is compelling evidence to suggest a beneficial role of lycopene in the prevention of prostate cancer. Evidence also is mounting in favor of lycopene in the prevention of other forms of cancer and of cardiovascular disease. It may also fight osteoporosis and age-related macular degeneration. It also may help prevent other diseases.

That's good news, and so is the fact that lycopene is part of many delicious foods you already enjoy. Let's take a look at a few recipes for brightening your menus while hopefully improving your health.

CHAPTER SIX

Now You're Cooking

Tasty Recipes for a Healthy Lifestyle

Good health can taste great. Here's a sample menu of a healthy meal that is low in fat and high in vitamins, antioxidants and lycopene:

Cocktail	Tomato juice or Bloody Mary
Soup	Tomato soup or vegetable soup with tomato
Main Course	Tuna or other fish (served with tomato-based seafood sauce)
	Broccoli or spinach
	Carrots
	Pasta with tomato sauce
	Multi-grain or whole wheat bread (with a cholesterol-reducing margarine)
Beverage	Red wine
Dessert	Fruit compote or yogurt
Beverage	Green tea

Recipes Rich in Lycopene

Beef and Vegetable Stir Fry

Ingredients:
- 2 cups (500 ml) hot cooked rice
- 1 pound (500 g) boneless beef sirloin
- 1 bag (16 oz./500 g) frozen mixed vegetables
- 1/2 tsp. (2 ml) ground ginger
- 1/3 cup (75 ml) College Inn beef broth
- 2 tbsp. (25 ml) soy sauce
- 2/3 cup (150 ml) Heinz Tomato Ketchup

In small bowl, combine ketchup, broth, soy sauce, and ginger; set aside. In large, nonstick skillet, quickly brown meat; remove. Add vegetables and ketchup mixture. Cover; simmer five to six minutes, or until vegetables are tender-crisp. Return beef to skillet; heat. Serve over rice.

Makes four servings.

Chicken Italia

Ingredients:
- 1 clove minced garlic
- 1 cup (250 ml) Heinz Tomato Ketchup
- 1 cup (250 ml) water
- 1 cup (250 ml) shredded mozzarella cheese
- 1 large, chopped tomato
- 1 medium, chopped onion
- 1 tbsp. (15 ml) vegetable oil
- 1/2 tsp. (2 ml) Italian seasoning
- 4 boneless chicken breast halves
- cooked pasta

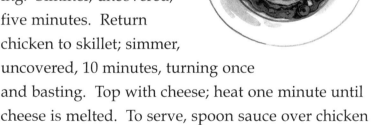

In large skillet, brown chicken in oil; remove and set aside. Sauté onion and garlic until tender. Add ketchup, water, tomato and seasoning. Simmer, uncovered, five minutes. Return chicken to skillet; simmer, uncovered, 10 minutes, turning once and basting. Top with cheese; heat one minute until cheese is melted. To serve, spoon sauce over chicken and pasta.

Makes four servings.

Honey Apple Barbeque Sauce

Ingredients:
- 1 cup (250 ml) Heinz Tomato Ketchup
- 1/4 tsp. (1 ml) ground cinnamon
- 2 tbsp. (30 ml) honey
- 2/3 cup (150 ml) applesauce

In small saucepan, combine ketchup, applesauce, honey, and cinnamon. Bring to a boil; reduce heat and simmer, uncovered, five minutes, stirring occasionally. Brush on chicken, pork, or turkey during last 10 minutes of grilling. Heat any remaining sauce to boiling; cook two minutes. Serve with grilled poultry or meat.

Makes 1-2/3 cups (380 ml).

Southwestern Pasta Salad

Ingredients:
- leaf lettuce
- shredded cheddar cheese
- 1 chopped fresh tomato
- 1 can drained kidney beans
- 1 can undrained corn
- 1 cup (250 ml) Heinz Tomato Ketchup
- 1 tbsp. (15 ml) taco seasoning mix
- 1/2 cup (125 ml) chopped red or green bell pepper
- 1/2 cup (125 ml) sliced black or green olives
- 1/2 cup (125 ml) sliced celery
- 1/2 cup (125 ml) sliced green onions
- 1/3 cup (75 ml) milk
- 1/4 cup (50 ml) mayonnaise
- 3 cups (750 ml) uncooked rotini

Cook pasta according to package directions. Drain and rinse; chill. In large bowl, combine pasta, beans, corn, tomato, bell pepper, celery, onions, and olives. For dressing, combine ketchup, mayonnaise and taco seasoning. Stir in milk. Add dressing to pasta mixture; toss to combine. Serve salad on lettuce. Sprinkle each serving with cheese.

Makes five to six servings.

TURKEY-BEAN TATER TOT CASSEROLE

Ingredients:
- 1 package (16 oz./500 g) Ore-Ida Tater Tots
- 1 can (16 oz./500 g) Heinz Baked Beans
- 1 can (16 oz./500 g) black beans, undrained
- 1 tsp. (5 ml) salt
- 1 pound (500 g) ground turkey
- 1 can (16 oz./500 g) cut green beans, undrained
- 1 can (15 oz./500 g) red kidney beans, undrained
- 1 large onion, chopped
- 1/2 cup (125 ml) Heinz Tomato Ketchup
- 1 can (15 oz./500 g) lima beans, undrained
- 6 tbsp. (90 ml) brown sugar
- 1 tbsp. (15 ml) Heinz White Vinegar
- 1-3 tsp. (5-15 ml) chili powder, optional

In a large nonstick skillet, brown turkey and onion until turkey is cooked. Drain lima and green beans, reserving liquid.

Add bean liquid, sugar, ketchup, vinegar, salt, and chili powder to skillet; bring to a boil. Meanwhile, combine lima, green, baked, kidney, and black beans in a 13-in. x 9-in. x 2-in. (330 mm x 230 mm x 50 mm) baking dish. Spoon turkey mixture over bean mixture. Bake, uncovered, at 350° F (175° C) for 40 minutes. Top with Tater Tots; bake an additional 30 minutes or until Tots are crisp.

Makes eight servings.

Hearty Potato Tomato Soup

Ingredients:
- 3 cups (750 ml) peeled, diced potatoes
- 1 cup (250 ml) finely diced celery
- 1/4 cup (50 ml) finely chopped onion
- 2 cups (500 ml) water
- 2-1/2 cups (625 ml) tomato juice
- 1/2 tsp. (2 ml) black pepper
- 1/3 cup (75 ml) table (18%) cream

Combine potatoes, celery, onion and water; boil gently, uncovered, until potatoes are soft. Mash potatoes in water. Stir in tomato juice and pepper; heat through. Just before serving, add cream and stir until hot; do not boil. Serve with croutons or toast.

Makes four servings.

No Fuss Cabbage Rolls

Ingredients:
- 4 cups (1 L) shredded cabbage
- 1 pound (500 g) extra lean ground beef*
- 1 large onion, finely chopped
- 1/2 tsp. (2 ml) salt
- 2/3 cup (150 ml) uncooked long grain rice
- 3-1/2 cups (875 ml) tomato juice
- 1/3 cup (75 ml) Heinz Chili Sauce
- 1/2 tsp. (2 ml) garlic powder

In large 10-cup (2.5 L) casserole, layer a third of the cabbage, half of each of the meat, onion, garlic powder, salt and rice. Pour one cup (250 ml) tomato juice over layers. Add a second layer of the six ingredients and then another cup of tomato juice. Top with remaining cabbage. Stir chili sauce into remaining tomato juice; pour over casserole. Bake covered, in 325° F (160° C) oven 1-1/2 to 2 hours. Serve with sour cream, if desired.

Makes eight servings.

*If using regular ground beef, brown and drain before layering in casserole.

Quick 'n' Easy Pita Pizza

Ingredients:
- 4 pita breads, 8 inches (20 cm)
- 2 cups (500 ml) shredded mozzarella cheese
- 1/4 cup (50 ml) each chopped green and red bell peppers
- 24 slices pepperoni

Pizza Sauce:
- 1 cup (250 ml) Heinz Tomato Ketchup
- 1 tsp. (5 ml) oregano
- 1 tsp. (5 ml) salt
- 1/2 tsp. (2 ml) black pepper
- 1 tsp. (5 ml) grated parmesan cheese

Combine all sauce ingredients; mix well.

For one pizza:
Spread each pita round with 1/4 cup (50 ml) sauce; top with mozzarella, peppers and pepperoni. Bake at 450° F (230° C) for 10 minutes, or until cheese melts.

Makes four pizzas.

Quick 'n' Easy Stir Fry

Ingredients:
- 2 tsp. (30 ml) vegetable oil, divided
- 1 pound (500 g) boneless pork or chicken, cut into strips or cubes
- 4 cups (1 L) broccoli pieces
- 1 onion, sliced
- 1 cup (250 ml) Heinz Chili Sauce
- 1/2 cup (125 ml) tomato juice
- 2 tsp. (10 ml) Worcestershire sauce
- 1 tsp. (5 ml) prepared horseradish
- 1/4 tsp. (1 ml) pepper

Heat 1 tbsp. (15 ml) oil in large skillet; brown meat. Add remaining oil, broccoli and onion; sauté lightly. Stir in remaining ingredients; cook about five minutes. Serve over two cups (500 ml) cooked tomato rice. (Prepare rice according to package directions, substituting tomato juice for half of the water.)

Makes four servings.

SWEET & SPICY SPAGHETTI SAUCE WITH MEAT

Ingredients:
- 1 pound (500 g) lean ground beef
- 2 tbsp. (25 ml) vegetable oil
- 2 cloves garlic, minced
- 1 medium onion, chopped
- 1 bottle (285 ml) Heinz Chili Sauce
- 2 cups (500 ml) tomato juice
- 2 tbsp. (25 ml) tomato paste
- 1 tsp. (5 ml) basil
- 1 tsp. (5 ml) oregano
- 1 tsp. (5 ml) salt
- 1 tsp. (5 ml) marjoram
- 1 bay leaf

In a 2 qt. (2 L) saucepan over medium heat in hot oil, brown ground beef, garlic and onion. Drain fat. Stir in chili sauce, tomato juice, tomato paste, and remaining ingredients. Reduce heat to low, partially cover and simmer sauce 35 to 45 minutes, stirring occasionally. Remove bay leaf before serving.

Makes four servings.

CHAPTER SEVEN

Q & A

SUMMING UP THE STORY OF LYCOPENE

Here are a few frequently asked questions and their answers.

WHAT IS LYCOPENE?

Lycopene, which gives red tomatoes their color, is one of a family of pigments called carotenoids, which occur naturally in fruits and vegetables. Other carotenoids include alpha- and beta-carotene, lutein, etc. Numerous studies suggest that antioxidants such as lycopene may actively inhibit the development of prostate, digestive tract, breast, lung and cervical cancer, as well as cardiovascular disease, diabetes, and age-related macular degeneration — the most common form of blindness for elderly people in the Western world.

Q & A

Does it prevent cancer?

Cancer risk is determined by many factors; however, diet is an important one. The importance of eating fresh and processed fruits and vegetables as part of a healthy diet has been well recognized for some time. Tomatoes and tomato products are rich in lycopene, a powerful antioxidant that picks up free radicals in the body, and can play a key role in that process. And while it is still too early to conclude that any single food can prevent cancer, the research to date is both promising and exciting.

How does it work?

Lycopene is an antioxidant that once absorbed by the body helps to protect cells and repair damaged cells. Antioxidants are compounds that fight free radicals in the body and have been shown to inhibit DNA oxidation that can lead to some cancers.

How can I get more lycopene?

The human body does not produce lycopene, but it's readily available through the diet. Minor sources include guava, rosehip, watermelon and pink grapefruit. About 85 percent of dietary lycopene comes from tomatoes and tomato products such as juice, soup, sauce, paste and ketchup. Research confirms that lycopene from tomatoes is absorbed much better into the bloodstream if it is first processed.

WHAT KIND OF BENEFITS CAN I GET FROM LYCOPENE?

As lycopene levels in the blood increase, the levels of oxidized compounds decrease. Growing medical evidence associates high intake of lycopene-rich tomato products with reduced risk of cancers of the lung, breast, prostate, cervix and digestive tract. For instance, eating tomato products regularly has been found to decrease the risk of cancer of the digestive tract among Italians. Lycopene also may help to prevent macular degenerative disease, the leading cause of blindness in people over the age of 65.

WHAT PROOF IS AVAILABLE THAT LYCOPENE HAS THESE BENEFITS?

In recent years, a number of studies have indicated that a lycopene-rich diet lowers the risk of certain chronic diseases such as cancer and heart disease, including:

- A human study conducted by the University of Toronto on dietary lycopene confirmed that it acts as an antioxidant. As lycopene levels in the blood go up, the levels of oxidized lipoprotein, protein and DNA compounds go down. This, in turn, helps to lower the risk of cancer and heart disease.

- A study of 47,894 men by the Harvard School of Medicine estimated that consuming tomato products twice a week, as opposed to never, was associated with a reduced risk of prostate cancer of up to 34 percent. Of 46 fruits and vegetables evaluated, only tomato products showed a measurable relationship with reduced prostate cancer risk.

- Research on breast, lung and endometrial cancer at Ben Gurion University and Soroka Medical Center in Israel shows that lycopene is even more effective than its cousins, alpha- and beta-carotene, in causing a delay in the cell cycle progression from one growth phase to the next.

- Another study, conducted by the University of North Carolina, compared fat samples from 1,379 American and European men who had suffered a heart attack with those of healthy men. It found that men with high levels of lycopene were half as likely to have had a heart attack as those with low levels of lycopene.

- Age-related macular degeneration (ARMD) is the most common form of blindness for elderly people in the Western world. Lycopene is the only micro-nutrient whose serum level is shown to be inversely related to the risk of ARMD.

CAN'T I GET THE SAME BENEFITS FROM EATING FRESH TOMATOES?

Yes, red tomatoes are rich in lycopene. However, cooking fresh tomatoes with a little oil will enhance the body's absorption of lycopene. Research confirms that the lycopene in tomatoes is converted by the temperature change involved in processing, which allows the body to absorb it more easily. A recent study showed that lycopene is absorbed 2.5 times better from tomato paste than from fresh tomatoes.

HOW MUCH DO I HAVE TO EAT TO MAKE A DIFFERENCE?

To date, no nutritional authority has published recommendations for lycopene intake. More research is needed before lycopene's full public health benefits can be determined and intake guidelines developed. However, based on recent evidence, many health professionals now advocate a diet rich in processed tomato products.

Processed tomato products should be part of the five to nine servings per day of the fruit and vegetable group suggested by food guidelines promoted in most industrialized countries.

ARE THERE PRODUCTS OTHER THAN TOMATOES THAT CONTAIN LYCOPENE?

Rosehip, pink grapefruit, guava, papaya and watermelon also contain lycopene; however, processed tomato products are usually the highest sources of dietary lycopene.

DOES ANY MEDICAL BODY OR ORGANIZATION ENDORSE LYCOPENE?

More detailed population studies of lycopene and wide-ranging clinical and biological research are needed before most health organizations can formally endorse lycopene for its health benefits. Several such studies are now underway in different parts of the world. Researchers hope to determine the role tomato products and lycopene play in disease prevention. However, because the early research indicates that consumption of tomatoes and processed tomato products — as part of a healthy lifestyle that includes a nutritious diet with from five to nine daily servings of fruits and vegetables — shows great promise in reducing the risk of several diseases, including heart disease and certain types of cancer, more and more medical professionals recommend the consumption of lycopene-rich tomato products.

WHAT OTHER RESEARCH IS BEING CONDUCTED?

Current studies are looking at the relationship between dietary lycopene, oxidative stress and cancer risk. The studies will further examine the role of lycopene as an antioxidant in preventing cancers of the breast, prostate, colon, cervix, lung and digestive tract, as well as cardiovascular disease and degenerative diseases of the eye, osteoporosis, diabetes and other diseases.

HOW CAN I GET THE RESULTS OF THE FUTURE STUDIES?

The Web site www.lycopene.org will provide ongoing information on lycopene and the research results of studies from around the globe.

Glossary

Adipose tissue: Connective tissue in which fat is stored.

Antioxidants: Substances that have the ability to inactivate harmful free radicals. There is growing scientific evidence that a diet high in antioxidants may protect against certain chronic diseases such as cancer, coronary heart disease, and cataracts. Substances in food with antioxidant activity that are not vitamins or minerals are sometimes referred to as phytochemicals. Lycopene in tomatoes is an example of a phytochemical with potent antioxidant activity.

Atherosclerosis: A condition in which the lining of the arteries becomes narrow. Caused by an accumulation of fat and other substances, it can lead to coronary heart disease, stroke, and other cardiovascular disorders.

Beta-carotene: The carotenoid in tomatoes with the most Vitamin A activity. It also has antioxidant activity. Once thought to be a major player in cancer prevention, recent scientific studies show less encouraging results, possibly because beta-carotene was studied alone rather than in association with other vitamins and antioxidants.

Botany: The branch of biology concerned with plants.

Calories: Calories are units of energy, commonly used to measure the amount of energy in food and also the amount of energy used by the body.

Carbohydrates: Substances made out of carbon, hydrogen and oxygen, usually sugars and starches. They are a good source of energy. Examples are cereals, breads, pastas, grains, and vegetables, such as potatoes.

Carotenoids: The source of Vitamin A activity in tomatoes. Carotenoids are plant pigments, responsible for the bright, rosy color of tomatoes. Carotenoids are fat-soluble, which means they are better absorbed in the presence of oil or fat. There are a number of different carotenoids in tomatoes, such as beta-carotene and lycopene.

Glossary

Cholesterol: A substance in the blood that helps produce hormones, transport nutrients in the bloodstream, and remove fatty waste products. Where cholesterol is associated with high levels of low-density lipoprotein (LDL), the buildup of fatty plaques on arteries can result. That buildup of plaque may contribute to cardiovascular disease.

Fiber: A mixture of indigestible carbohydrates found in plant foods. It does not supply calories or nutrients, but aids in digestion and elimination. Tomatoes are a source of fiber; people who eat diets high in fiber have a lowered risk of heart disease. Fiber also may protect against some cancers.

Folic Acid: This is a B vitamin that also is known as folacin and folate. It is important in a number of bodily processes, including the production of red blood cells and the development of a fetus.

Free radicals: Highly reactive oxygen byproducts created by normal cell metabolism. Free radicals lack electrons and try to steal them from other molecules, damaging them. This damage is thought to be a fundamental cause of many degenerative diseases and the aging process. If free radicals attack the molecules involved in normal cellular reproduction, cells may become cancerous. Free radicals can damage the molecules responsible for moving cholesterol through the bloodstream, resulting in the buildup of plaque in the arteries.

Homocysteine: An amino acid. Some research links high levels of this substance with an increased incidence of heart disease.

Horticulture: The study of growing fruits, vegetables, flowers, and other plants.

Lycopene: The red pigment that gives tomatoes their color, and the predominant carotenoid in tomatoes. Lycopene does not convert to Vitamin A, but may have enormous significance in disease prevention due to its potent antioxidant activity. Lycopene is the most abundant carotenoid in human blood and tissues. Tomatoes are the primary source of lycopene in our diet.

Macular degeneration: A disease in which nerve tissue in the retina deteriorates, leading to gradual loss of sight. It is commonly associated with advancing age.

Niacin: Niacin, also called Vitamin B3, is important in many bodily processes, including breaking down food into energy. It has health benefits for the skin, digestive tract and nerves.

Oligosaccharides: Non-digestible oligosaccharides are a kind of carbohydrate that is not digested or absorbed by the body. They may help produce healthful bacteria in the digestive tract.

Osteoporosis: A disease in which bones become thinner and weaker; people suffering from osteoporosis are more likely to suffer broken bones.

Oxidation: A chemical reaction involving oxygen. Many scientists believe that, in the body, the oxidation process may create free radicals and damage cells, leading to disease.

Phytochemicals: Hundreds of substances produced naturally by plants to protect themselves from disease. The exact role phytochemicals play in promoting human health is still under investigation, but many phytochemicals have antioxidant activity.

Potassium: Potassium is a mineral that works with sodium to aid the proper functioning of muscles, including the heart.

Proteins: Molecules made up of amino acids. Proteins play many vital roles in the body, including growth and development, cell repair, antibody production, and the production of important chemicals.

Retinol: Retinol is the form of Vitamin A that is derived from animal sources. Carotenoids are the precursors of Vitamin A found in plants.

Vitamins: Essential substances that must be consumed because the body is unable to manufacture them. They are required to maintain health and normal body functions; consuming insufficient amounts may cause disease. Tomatoes are a significant source of Vitamin A and Vitamin C.

Glossary

Vitamin A: Vitamin A is essential for vision, normal growth, reproduction, and a healthy immune system. There are two types of Vitamin A — retinoids (preformed Vitamin A found in foods of animal origin) and carotenoids (found in foods of plant origin and converted into Vitamin A). A medium tomato supplies 20 percent of our daily value for Vitamin A.

Vitamin C: Also referred to as ascorbic acid, Vitamin C plays a vital role in combating infection, keeping gums healthy and healing wounds. Vitamin C also is involved in bone health and in regulating blood pressure. One medium tomato meets 40 percent of our daily need for Vitamin C. The vitamin also functions as an antioxidant and may have an additional role in chronic disease prevention, such as cancer and heart disease.

Information in the above glossary includes terms from the Tomato Nutrition Glossary of the Florida Tomato Committee, Copyright 2000, www.floridatomatoes.org/nutrition.html, used with permission from the Florida Tomato Committee.

Sources

Foreword
For more information on prostate cancer, go to www.cdc.gov/cancer/prostate/prostate.htm

Chapter One

American Cancer Society, "Prevention and Risk Factors," www3.cancer.org/cancerinfo/load_cont.asp?st-pr&ct-1&language=english

American Dietetic Association, "Position of The American Dietetic Association: Phytochemicals and Functional Foods," *Journal of the American Dietetic Association*, 1995, 95:493

American Heart Association, Nutrition Committee, "Dietary Guidelines for Healthy American Adults," *Circulation*, 1996, 94:1795-1800

American Medical Association, "AMA Health Insight," www.ama-assn.org/insight/spec_con/patient/pat071.pdf

Arab, Lenore, and Steck, Susan, "Lycopene and Cardiovascular Disease," *The American Journal of Clinical Nutrition*, 71:6, 1691S-1695S, June 2000

Food and Nutrition Science Alliance, "Up to One-Third of All Cancer Cases May Be Prevented by Healthy Diets and Exercise, Notes FANSA," Jan. 11, 2000

Giovannuccci, E., et al, "Intake of Carotenoids and Retinol in Relation to Risk of Prostate Cancer," *Journal of the National Cancer Institute*, 1995, 87:1767-1776

International Food Information Council, "Background on Functional Foods," December 1999, Washington, DC, www.ificinfo.health.org/qanda/qafunctional.htm

SOURCES

Kurtzweil, Paula, "An FDA Guide to Dietary Supplements," *FDA Consumer*, U.S. Food and Drug Administration, September-October 1998, revised January 1999; vm.cfsan.fda.gov/'dms/fdsupplhtml

McBride, Judy, "High-ORAC Foods May Slow Aging," *News from the USDA Agricultural Research Service*, www.ars.usda.gov/is/pr/1999/990208.htm

National Cancer Institute, "Risk Factors: Diet and Cancer Risk," rex.nci.nih.gov/NCI_Pub_Interface/raterisk/risks73.html

Rudge, Kate, "Scientific Food with Protective Benefits," International Food Information Service, February 1999, (See "Hot Topics" at www.ifis.org)

Snodderly, D.M., "Evidence for Protection Against Age-Related Macular Degeneration by Carotenoids and Antioxidant Vitamins," *The American Journal of Clinical Nutrition*, 1995, 62:1448S-1461S

Taylor, A., et al, "Relations Among Aging, Antioxidant Status, and Cataract," *The American Journal of Clinical Nutrition*, 1995, 62:1439S-1447S

Tribble, Diane, for the Nutrition Committee of the American Heart Association, "Antioxidant Consumption and Risk of Coronary Heart Disease," *Circulation*, 1999, 99:591-595

U.S. Department of Health and Human Services, "National Nutrition Summit 2000: Highlights of HHS Initiatives on Nutrition and Physical Activity," May 30, 2000

U.S. Food and Drug Administration, "Fruits and Vegetables: Eating Your Way to 5 A Day," www.pueblo.gsa.gov/cic_text/food/eating5aday/297_five.html

CHAPTER TWO

Andersen, Craig R., "Tomatoes," University of Arkansas, Division of Agriculture, Cooperative Extension Service, www.uaex.edu/Other_Areas/publications/HTML/FSA-6017.asp

California Tomato Growers Association (CTGA) Web site, www.ctga.org/html/html/FastFacts.html

Castleman, Elisabeth Glascon, "Tomato in America," Oct. 28, 2000; AboutFood Web site, www.aboutfood.co.uk/articles/content/article-222.html

Columbia Encyclopedia: Sixth Edition; 2000, www.bartleby.com/65/to/tomato/html

Cutler, Karan Davis, "From Wolf Peach to Outer Space: Tomato History & Lore," The Brooklyn Botanic Garden Web site, www.bbg.org/gardening/kitchen/tomatoes/cutler.html

National Garden Bureau, "Year of the Tomato," www.ngb.org/5/a20.asp

Smith, Andrew F., *Pure Ketchup*; University of South Carolina Press, 1996, p.17-27

Winter, Norman, "Tomatoes Rank No. 1 in Mississippi Gardens," Office of Agricultural Communications, Mississippi State University, April 2, 1998 (Available at Web site, www.msucares.com/news/print/lgnews/msgnews/sg980402.htm)

CHAPTER THREE

Andersen, Craig R. , "Tomatoes," University of Arkansas, Division of Agriculture, Cooperative Extension Service, www.uaex.edu/Other_Areas/publications/HTML/FSA-6017.asp

Burpee Seeds & Plants Web site, www.burpee.com

California Tomato Growers Association (CTGA) Web site, www.ctga.org/html/html/FastFacts.html

Sources

Castleman, Elisabeth Glascon, "Tomato in America," Oct. 28, 2000; AboutFood Web site, www.aboutfood.co.uk/articles/content/article-222.html

Cutler, Karan Davis, "From Wolf Peach to Outer Space: Tomato History & Lore," The Brooklyn Botanic Garden Web site, www.bbg.org/gardening/kitchen/tomatoes/cutler.html

Economic Research Service, U.S. Department of Agriculture, "Vegetables and Specialties Situation and Outlook Yearbook," VGS-281, July 2000

Encyclopedia Britannica,"Solanaceae," www.britannica.com/bcom/eb/article/0/0,5716,74730+1+72825,00.html?query=tomatoes

Lerner, B. Rosie, "1998 Is the Year of the Tomato," Horticulture and Landscape Architecture Department, Purdue University, Web site, www.hort.purdue.edu/ext/98tomato.html

Lucier, Gary, "Fresh-Market Tomato Industry Trends," *The Tomato Magazine*, August 2000, www.freshcut.com/page.cfm?userdate=2000-08-01%2000:00:00&magazine=5

National Garden Bureau, "Year of the Tomato," www.ngb.org/scripts/view_article.pl?id=20

Nix v. Hedden, 149 U.S. 304 (1893), www.caselaw.lp.findlaw.com/scripts/getcase.pl?court=us&vol=149&invol=304

"Tomato: Fruit or Vegetable?," University of Illinois, College of Agricultural, Consumer and Environmental Sciences, Cooperative Extension Service, Horticulture Solutions Series, www.ag.uiuc.edu/~robsond/solutions/horticulture/docs/tomato.html

U.S. Department of Agriculture Nutrient Database for Standard Reference, Release 13, November 1999, www.nal.usda.gov/fnic/cgi-bin/list_nut.pl

WSU Cooperative Extension, "Tomato Varieties," *Gardening in Western Washington*, Washington State University, www.gardening.wsu.edu/library/vege008/vege008.htm

CHAPTER FOUR

Charles, M.R., "The Tomato," *Scientific American*, 1978, 239:76-87

Kurtzweil, Paula, "Scouting for Sodium And Other Nutrients Important to Blood Pressure," United States Food and Drug Administration, *FDA Consumer*, September 1994, rev. September 1995, at: www.vm.cfsan.fda.gov/~dms/fdsodium.html

Nachbar, M.S., Oppenheim, "Lectins in the United States Diet: A Survey of Lectins in Commonly Consumed Foods and a Review of the Literature," *The American Journal of Clinical Nutrition*, 1980, 33:2338-2345

National Agricultural Laboratory, United States Department of Agriculture, www.nal.usda.gov/fnic/cgi-bin/lisy_nut.pl

Shi, J. Le Maguer, M., "Lycopene in Tomatoes: Chemical and Physical Properties Affected by Food Processing," *Critical Reviews in Food Science and Nutrition*, 2000, 40:1-42

Spiegel, J.E., et al, "Safety and Benefits of Froctooligosaccharides as Food Ingredients," *Food Technology*, 1994, 1:85-89

United States Department of Agriculture, "Nutrition and Your Health: Dietary Guidelines for Americans," USDA fifth ed., 2000

SOURCES

CHAPTER FIVE

For more information and complete sources, see:

Agarwal, Sanjiv, and Rao, Venket, "Tomato Lycopene and Its Role in Human Health and Chronic Diseases," *Canadian Medical Association Journal*, Sept. 19, 2000, 163(6), 739-44

For more information on lycopene, diabetes and ARMD, see:

Ford, E.S., et al, "Diabetes Mellitus and Serum Carotenoids: Findings from the Third National Health and Nutrition Examination Survey," *American Journal of Epidemiology*, 149(2): 168-176

Mares-Perlman, J.A., et al, "Serum Antioxidants and Age-Related Macular Degeneration in a Population-based Case-Control Study," *Archives of Ophthalmology*, December 1995, 113(12):1518-23

Index

A
Acid-base balance, 25
Adipose tissue, 38, 62
  heart attacks, antioxidant levels (relationship), 38
Adrenal gland, 32
Age-matched control subjects, 36
Age-related macular degeneration (ARMD), 5, 28, 39–40, 54, 58
  fighting, 42
Agglutination activity, 29
Alpha-carotene, 54, 57
American Cancer Society, 3
American Heart Association, 3
American Medical Association (AMA), 3
Amino acids, 26
Anorexia, 26
Antioxidants, 5-8
  See Dietary antioxidants
  effects. *See* Lycopene
  examination, 30
  interaction. *See* Disease
  levels, relationship. *See also* Cancer; Heart; Oxidative damage
Apple. *See* Golden apple of love (poma amoris/ pomme d'amour), 9–10
Arthritis, 5
Atherosclerosis, 62
  development/progression, 37

B
B vitamins, 26, 63
Bacteria. *See* Intestinal tract
  fighting, 29
  nourishment. *See* Colon
Beefsteak tomatoes, 17
Belladonna, 11
Beta-carotene, 7, 24, 54, 57, 62
Bleeding gums, 24
Blindness, 24, 40, 54. *See also* Night blindness
  cause, 56
  form, 58
Blood
  clots, prevention, 28
  lycopene levels, 36
    increase, 56
    reduction, 38
  pressure, 4
Body lipids, 28
Bone cells, activity, 40
Breast cancer, 34
  prevention, 60
  research, 57
Broccoli, 2, 43, 52

C
Cabbage, 19, 25
Calcium, 23
Calcium-fortified orange juice, 4
Cancer. *See* Breast cancer; Prostate cancer
  antioxidants, usage, 33–35
  causing, 28
  cells, proliferation, 37
  incidence, 35
  prevention. *See* Colon
    lycopene usage, 55. *See also* Chemically induced cancer; Spontaneous cancer

INDEX

reduction, 28. *See* also
  Digestive tract cancers
risk, 42, 55
  oxidative stress, 37
  reduction, 37, 56
  relationship, 60
  types, 60
Carbohydrate-binding protein, 29
Carbohydrates, 62
Cardiovascular disease, 54
  fighting, 7
  prevention, 28, 39
  protection, 38
  risk, 39, 42
  reduction, 38
Carotenoids, 28, 54, 62–63
  beneficial role, indirect evidence, 38
  conversion. *See* Vitamin A
  demonstration, 24, 28
  effect, 34
Carrots, 19, 25, 43
Cauliflower, 19
Cayenne pepper, 14
Celery, 19, 47, 49
Cells. *See* Rodent osteoclast cells
  activity. *See* Bone cells
  damage, 28
  development, 33
  genetic alteration, 33
  membranes, nutrient movement, 25–26
  proliferation, 33. *See* also Cancer
Cervical cancer (development), inhibition, 54
Cervix cancer
  prevention, 60
  risk reduction, 56

Chemically induced cancer (prevention), lycopene usage, 34
Cherry tomatoes, 17
Cholesterol, 63
  carriers, 37
  reduction, 21, 38
Chronic diseases, 40, 42
  risk reduction, 56
Citrus fruits, 24
Clinical intervention studies, 39
Colon
  bacteria nourishment, 28
  cancer, prevention, 60
Control subjects.
  See Age-matched control subjects
Coronary artery disease, rate, 38
Cramps, 26
Cucumbers, 19

D

Daily diet, lycopene usage, 41–42
Death, causes, 4
Degenerative diseases, 24
Depression, 5
Dessert, 19
Determinate plants, indeterminate plants (contrast), 16
Diabetes, 5, 40, 54
  reduction, 28
Diet. *See* Daily diet; Lycopene-rich diet
  choice, 21
Dietary antioxidants, 37
Dietary lycopene, 37, 56, 59
  level, 42
  relationship, 60
Digestive tract cancers
  development, inhibition, 54

prevention, 60
reduction, 34
risk, reduction, 56
Digitalis, 5
Disease. *See* Chronic disease
   antioxidants, interaction, 39–41
   prevention, 1. *See also*
   Cardiovascular disease
   protection. *See* Inflammatory
   intestinal/bowel diseases
   rate. *See* Coronary artery
   disease reduction. *See* Heart
   risk reduction, 59–60. *See also*
   Cardiovascular disease
Disease-fighting foods, 4–5
DNA, 28, 30
   compounds, decrease, 57
   damage, 33
   oxidation, inhibition, 55
   oxidative damage, prevention, 37
Double bonds, 31

E
Edible wolf peach.
   See Lycopersicon esculentum
Eggplant, 14
Electrolyte, 25
Endometrial cancer, research, 57
Environmental factors, 6
Epidemiological studies, 33–35, 38

F
Fats, 28, 30
FDA. *See* U.S. Food and Drug
   Administration
Fiber, 63
   sources, 22
Fish, 19, 27, 43
Folic acid, 23, 26, 63
   See Pregnant women

intake, amount, 27
Food Pyramid, 22
Free radicals, 5-6, 28, 30, 63
   effect, 31, 37
   fighting, 55
Fresh tomatoes, benefits
   (lycopene comparison), 58
Fruits, 1, 2, 4, 8, 22, 27, 54. *See
   also* Citrus fruits; Red fruits
   compote, 43
   evaluation, 57
   servings, 59
Functional components.
   See Tomatoes
Functional foods, 4-5

G
Garlic, 27, 45, 53
   powder, 50
Genetic materials, 28
Ginger, 44
Glucose tolerance, 40
Golden apple, 9
Grains, 2. *See also* Whole grains
Green tea, 27, 43
Ground beef. *See* Lean ground
   beef
Guava, 55. *See also* Pink guava
   lycopene content, 59

H
Harvard School of Medicine, 7, 57
Health benefits. *See* Tomatoes
Heart
   attacks
      reduction, 2
      relationship.
      See Adipose tissue
      risk increase, 38
      suffering, 57

conditions, 5
disease, 5
   reduction, 27, 28, 56, 60
protection, antioxidants
   usage, 37–39
Heinz, 44-48, 50-53
High blood pressure, 4
   reduction, 26
High-risk population, 38, 39
Homocysteine, 26, 63
   amount, reduction, 27
Horticulture, 63

I

Immune functions, 25
Immune response,
   enhancement, 37
Immune system, boosting, 29
Indeterminate plants, contrast.
   See Determinate plants
Infections, prevention, 25
Inflammatory intestinal/
   bowel diseases, protection, 29
Initiation stage, 33
Intestinal enzymes, 28
Intestinal tract, bacteria, 27
Iron, absorption, 24

J

Jefferson, Thomas, 10
Johnson, Robert Gibbon, 11–12
Joints, soreness, 24

K

Ketchup, 12, 16, 36, 56
   amount, 42
   (Heinz), 44–48, 51
Kitjap, 12

L

LDL. *See* Low-density
   lipoprotein
Lettuce, 19, 25
Lifestyle factors, 2
Lipids, 28, 30. *See also* Body
   lipids oxidation, reduction, 41
   oxidative damage, prevention, 37
Lipoprotein
   decrease. *See* Oxidized
   lipoprotein
   oxidation. *See* Low-density
   lipoprotein
Liver, 32
Low-density lipoprotein
   (LDL), 63
   oxidation, 37
Lung cancer, 25
   development, inhibition, 54
   prevention, 60
   research, 57
   risk, reduction, 56
Lutein, 54
Lycopene, 63. *See also*
   Dietary lycopene
   absorption, 41, 58
   antioxidant effects, 37
   beneficial role. *See* Prostate
   cancer
   benefits, 41, 56
      proof, 56–58
   bioavailability, 31
   capsules, 41
   comparison. *See* Fresh
   tomatoes
   components, 27
   consumption, 7
   content. *See* Guava; Papaya;
   Pink grapefruit; Rosehip;
   Watermelons

explanation, 54
intake, 41-42, 58-59
　levels, 42
　lessons, 30
　levels. *See* Blood; Serum lycopene levels
　medical/organizational endorsement, 59-60
　recommended intake, 58-59
　research, 60
　results, obtaining, 60
　role, epidemiological evidence, 38-39
　story, summary, 54
　usage. *See* Cancer; Daily diet; Recipes increase, 55-56
Lycopene-rich diet, 56
Lycopene-rich tomato products, intake, 56, 60
Lycopersicon esculentum (edible wolf peach), 14

M
Macular degeneration, 64.
　See also Age-related macular degeneration disease, prevention, 56
Magnesium, 23, 26
Maturity date. *See* Tomatoes
Meat, 10, 19, 22
Mediterranean diet, 2, 34
Mental confusion, 26
Metastasis, 33
Micro-nutrient, 58
Minerals, 26
　sources, 22
Muscle
　contraction, 26
　weakness, 26

N
National Cancer Institute, 3
Nerve conduction, 26
Neural tube defects, risk reduction, 26
Niacin, 64
Night blindness, 24
Nightshade, 10
Non-digestible oligosaccharides, 64

O
Oligosaccharides, 27, 28, 64
　See also Non-digestible oligosaccharides
Olive oil, 2, 34
Onions, 18, 25, 45, 48-49, 52-53
Oranges, 24, 25
Osteoclast cells. *See* Rodent osteoclast cells
Osteoporosis, 5, 40, 64
　fighting, 42
　prevention, 4
Oxidation
　inhibition. *See* DNA
　reduction. *See* Lipids
　signs, 36, 41
Oxidative damage
　inhibition, 37
　prevention. *See* DNA; Lipids; Proteins
　reduction, 30
　　antioxidant usage, 37
　　relationship, 40
Oxidative stress, 42. *See also* Cancer
　reduction, 36
　relationship, 60
Oxidized lipoprotein, decrease, 56-57

Index

P
Papaya, lycopene content, 59
Parsnips, 19
Peach. *See* Wolf peach
Pear tomatoes, 17
Peas, 19
Phytochemicals, 5, 64
Pink grapefruit, 30, 36, 55
   lycopene content, 59
Pink guava, 30
Plant chemicals, 5
Plaque, 63
Plasma LDL levels, 38
Plum tomatoes, 17
Poma amoris. *See* Apple
Pomme d'amour. *See* Apple
Pomodoro, 9
Potassium, 23, 64
   content, 25–26
Potatoes, 14, 19, 25, 49
Pregnant women,
   folic acid importance, 26–27
Processed tomato products, 8, 31, 58
Progression stage, 33
Prostate, 32
Prostate cancer, 34–37
   development, inhibition, 54
   lycopene, beneficial role, 42
   patients, 36
   prevention, 42
   risk reduction, 7, 35, 56–57
Prostate specific antigen (PSA), 36
Proteins, 30, 64. *See also*
   Carbohydrate-binding protein
   levels, decrease, 57
   oxidation. See Low-density lipoprotein
   oxidative damage, prevention, 37

PSA. *See* Prostate specific antigen

Q
Quinine, 5

R
Raw tomato, 36
Red fruits, 30
Red wine, 27, 43
Refrigeration, 10
Retinol, 64
Rodent osteoclast cells, 40
Rosehip, 55
   lycopene content, 59

S
Saturated fat
   levels, 2
   reduction, 21
Serum level, 58
Serum lycopene levels, 41
Smoking, 6
Solanaceae, 14
Soroka Medical Center, 57
Soybeans, 27
Spontaneous cancer
   (prevention), lycopene usage, 34
Squashes, 19
Standard tomatoes, 17
Starches, 10, 22
Sugars. *See* Brown sugar
   intake moderation, 21
Sweet corn, 25
Sweet potatoes, 25

T

Tabasco pepper, 14
Tea. *See* Green tea
Testes, 32
Tissue culture studies, 33
Tomatl, 9
Tomato-based products, 30, 35
Tomatoes. *See* Beefsteak tomatoes; Cherry tomatoes; Pear tomatoes; Plum tomatoes; Raw tomato; Standard tomatoes
   benefits. *See* Fresh tomatoes
   color, 15–16
   consumption, 59
   essence, 23
   flavor, 17–18
   fruit/vegetable controversy, 18–19
   functional components, 27–29
   health benefits, 21
   history, 9-13
   intake, 34
   juice, 2, 32, 36, 43, 49, 52–53, 55
   maturity date, 17
   nutrients, 26–27
   origins, 9
   paste, 36, 53, 55–56
   popularity, 20
   processing, 16–17
   products, 13, 17, 23, 29, 38, 42, 55, 59. *See also* Processed tomato products
   intake. *See* Lycopene-rich tomato products
   ripeness, 16–17
   sauce, 36, 55
   shape, 17
   size, 15
   soup, 36, 43, 55. *See also* Hearty potato tomato soup
   storage, 16–17
   understanding, 14
   usage, 9
   varieties, 15–18
Tomato-harvesting machines, refinement, 12
Total fat, moderation, 21
Tumor, regression, 37
Turnips, 19

U

University of North Carolina, 7, 57
University of Toronto, 56
University of Wisconsin, 40
U.S. Department of Health and Human Services, 3
U.S. Food and Drug Administration (FDA), 3
U.S. Supreme Court, 19

V

Vegetables, 2, 4, 8, 22, 27, 30, 34, 54
   evaluation, 57
   fruit, controversy. *See* Tomatoes
   intake, 27
   oil, 45, 52, 53
   servings, 59
Vitamin A, 7, 23, 65
   carotenoids, conversion, 27–28
   content, 24–25
Vitamin B1, 23
Vitamin B2, 23
Vitamin B3, 64
Vitamin C, 4, 7, 65
   content, 23–24
Vitamin E, 7, 23, 32
Vitamins, 64. *See also* B vitamins
   sources, 22

W

Walnuts, 12
Watermelons, 30, 36, 55
   lycopene content, 59
Whole grains, 27
Whole wheat bread, 43
Wine. *See* Red wine
Wolf peach, 10, 11. *See also*
   Lycopersicon esculentum

Z

Zinc, absorption, 24

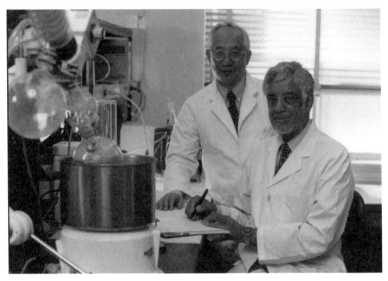

David Yeung, Ph.D., (left) and Venket Rao, Ph.D., in the laboratory.

DAVID YEUNG, PH.D.

David Yeung, Ph.D., is the Director, Corporate Nutrition, H.J. Heinz Company. He received his doctorate degree from the Department of Nutritional Sciences, Faculty of Medicine, University of Toronto.

He was an associate professor in Applied Human Nutrition at the University of Guelph, Ontario, before joining the H.J. Heinz Company of Canada. Dr. Yeung remains academically active. He is an Associate Professor in the Department of Nutritional Sciences, University of Toronto, and has been an adjunct and honorary professor in universities in Canada and the People's Republic of China.

Dr. Yeung has published extensively in refereed scientific journals, and he has served on numerous scientific committees in Canada and the U.S.

Dr. Yeung has extensive international experience. He has established nutrition education programs in Australia, Canada, China, the Czech Republic, Hungary, India, Poland, Spain, Thailand, and Russia. He has served as consultant to the Food and Agriculture Organization (FAO), The Micronutrients Initiatives (MI), and the U.S. Agency for International Development (USAID).

In 1997, Dr. Yeung received the Earle Willard McHenry Award from the Canadian Society of Nutritional Sciences for distinguished service in nutrition.

VENKET RAO, PH.D.

Venket Rao, Ph.D., obtained his M.S. and Ph.D. in Food Science from Oregon State University. Dr. Rao is a full professor in the Department of Nutritional Sciences, Faculty of Medicine, University of Toronto. He also is the Director of the Program in Food Safety. He is a member of the Canadian Federation of Biological Sciences, the Society of Toxicology of Canada, and the Bifidous Foundation of Japan.

Dr. Rao's research has established a major focus in the area of diet and cancer with particular emphasis on the role of phytochemicals in human nutrition and health. More recently, he has been investigating the role of oxidative stress and antioxidants in the causation and prevention of chronic diseases. He has studied the role of tomatoes and lycopene in human health extensively and has delivered lectures on this topic nationally and internationally. He has published extensively in scientific journals and participated in many national and international scientific conferences.

Dr. Rao is a member of the Provincial and National Expert Committees in Canada in the areas of food safety and agriculture. He is a member of the National Steering Committee to develop policy guidelines for the Safety of Raw Foods of Animal Origin. He is very active in the Department of Nutritional Sciences as a teacher, research supervisor and as the Undergraduate Coordinator of the Nutritional Sciences Specialist Program. He is frequently sought by the international media for commentary on the subjects of food safety, nutrition and health.